Langdon Frothingham

Laboratory Guide for the Bacteriologist

Langdon Frothingham

Laboratory Guide for the Bacteriologist

ISBN/EAN: 9783742831859

Manufactured in Europe, USA, Canada, Australia, Japa

Cover: Foto ©Lupo / pixelio.de

Manufactured and distributed by brebook publishing software
(www.brebook.com)

Langdon Frothingham

Laboratory Guide for the Bacteriologist

FOR THE

BACTERIOLOGIST

BY

LANGDON FROTHINGHAM, M. D. V.

ASSISTANT IN BACTERIOLOGY AND VETERINARY SCIENCE, SHEFFIELD
SCIENTIFIC SCHOOL, YALE UNIVERSITY.

ILLUSTRATED

PHILADELPHIA

W. B. SAUNDERS

925 WALNUT STREET.

1895.

CONTENTS.

(4)

PREFACE.

The following technical methods, arranged as simply and concisely as possible, are especially intended for convenience in laboratory work. One constantly wishes and uses the methods herein enumerated, and for the same must refer to the large text-books. It is to avoid this longer search, except for details, that the following scheme is published—a scheme which the writer adopted some years ago for his own convenience, and which he sincerely hopes others may also find a useful desk companion. Before describing the different methods, there are mentioned a few ways by which the work may be much accelerated—ways probably known to and practised by many, but not, perhaps, to all.

(ⴺ)

1. BACTERIOLOGICAL TECHNIQUE.

Of paramount importance in bacteriological technique is rapid work associated with the best possible results. In preparing, staining, and mounting cover-glass preparations much valuable time is too often wasted, and if this can be reduced to a minimum we are in many ways the gainers. On account of this loss of time the older method of making cover-glass preparations—by placing the material to be examined upon a cover-slip and pressing another slip upon it, staining them in a watch-glass with staining fluids made up when desired by adding a few drops of a concentrated alcoholic solution of the stain to be used to water or to aniline water, and mounting at once in Canada balsam—has greatly fallen into disuse.

By far the larger portion of cover-glass preparations made, are prepared purely and simply for the purpose of diagnosis; it is therefore ordinarily a useless waste of cover-slips to make two preparations from the same material, especially as such preparations are frequently much too thick to be considered beautiful or even worthy of permanent mounting. Similarly it is evident that it is needless to mount at once in Canada balsam, for cover-glass preparations are invariably thrown away after a short microscopical examination, not because the preparations are poor, but rather because they were made only for diagnosis, which having been accomplished they are only in the rarest cases of further use. Moreover, after mounting in balsam one should properly wait until the balsam is dry before examining in oil, or run the risk of making an unsightly preparation; here again much time is lost. Furthermore, the staining may be greatly accelerated. It is seldom necessary to stain in the watch-glass or to make up one's staining fluids as required; the fluids for ordinary staining should always be ready for use. The staining is best and simplest performed upon the cover-glass, after which the preparation may be mounted and at once examined in water. It is then a simple matter, if desired,

7

to remove the slip and to mount it permanently. It is particularly in the line of work above noted that much valuable time may be saved. The culture technique cannot greatly be accelerated, excepting in a few instances.

The principal object, then, to be aimed at is to gain as much time as possible, provided the best results are also obtained. For the first purpose everything that is necessary to work with must be within easy reach of the operator's hands, and for ordinary work he should never be obliged to leave his seat. The following description of his desk may, therefore, not be inappropriate.

LABORATORY DESK.—It will be found an invaluable aid, in all microscopic work, to have the desk covered with a large glass plate, perhaps 2 feet long by 17 inches wide. It will be advantageous if the glass plate is let into the woodwork of the desk. A working surface is thus obtained which has many advantages, one of the most important being its great cleanliness. This surface, however, may vastly be improved if one-half of the glass plate (from left to right) is painted jet-black, and the other half pure white, the painted side, of course, being placed downward. As it is sometimes difficult to obtain a pure white paint a piece of white paper of suitable size may be substituted. The advantage of a pure black-and-white background are obvious to anyone who has done much microscopic work. Unstained preparations, or sections, for instance, in the watch-glass, or upon the slide, stand out very distinctly upon the black side and stained ones upon the white side; in the same way different colonies upon the plate are seen to better advantage; the black surface, again, is particularly useful in selecting the best portions of tuberculous sputum for examination, etc. In fact, it will be found exceedingly practical in innumerable ways.

About 2 feet in front of the operator there should be placed three vessels—tumblers, for instance. One of these tumblers, containing a little cotton in the bottom, is used principally for holding three platinum needles, one straight, one with a large loop, and one with a small loop—a hooked and a flat needle, which are often useful, may be added if desired. This tumbler is a convenient place also to keep such articles as steel and fine glass needles for handling sections, a pair of scissors, forceps, etc. The other two tumblers are each filled daily with fresh water, the use of which will be apparent later.

On a line with the tumblers, or better still, on a small slightly-raised shelf behind them, should be placed several small bottles containing the fluids ordinarily used for staining bacteria. There are now several bottles used especially for this purpose, some being furnished with pipettes of different forms, with other means for transferring the stain to the cover-glass. Any small (2-ounce), firmly-standing bottle, however, through the cork of which passes a glass tube drawn out below, answers every demand. For ordinary work there should be five such bottles, each filled with one of the following staining fluids: Methylene-blue, Gentian-violet, Fuchsin, Ziehl's carbol-fuchsin solution and Gabbet's solution. Although the latter often fails to stain well, it nevertheless is an excellent decolorizer, and in the hands of an expert is admirable for making a rapid diagnosis of tuberculous sputum. To these stains may be added any other desired stain, such as Bismarck-brown, Loeffler's solution, etc. The usual staining fluids (Methylene-blue, Gentian-violet, Fuchsin) prepared as under I (foot-note 2 a) will not only give excellent staining results, but will also keep indefinitely.

Upon the desk there should also be a small bottle of cedar-oil, from which a small drop may quickly be transferred to the slide without necessitating the use of more than one hand. Within easy reach may be hung a bunch of filter-papers cut into strips, say 1.5 inches broad by 6 inches long. On a shelf above the desk may be placed a large bottle of distilled water, from which a rubber tube descends close to the hand; the tube is closed near its lower end with a Mohr pinch-cock (Fig. 1). This is an exceedingly convenient arrangement also for the corrosive-sublimate bottle. The desk is now in readiness, and should always be so for ordinary work, which must necessarily be much accelerated since everything that is desired is within reach.

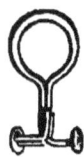

Fig. 1.

If there is any one thing the bacteriologist has to do more than another it is perhaps to make cover-glass preparations, especially if he is working upon any special organism. Although it may seem a simple matter to make such preparations, anyone who has had charge of students knows some of the difficulties to be surmounted—that is, if their results can be taken as criteria. Indeed, it is by no means so seldom that men of experience have difficulty in preparing what might be considered worthy specimens.

There will, therefore, be described rather minutely a well-known, very simple, and rapid method of preparing, staining, and mounting a cover-glass preparation.

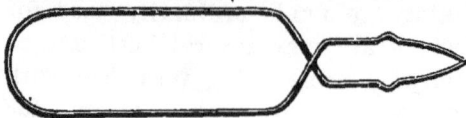

Fig. 2.—Cornet's Double-spring Forcep.

The well-cleaned glass is held between the thumb and fore-finger of the left hand. (A more convenient method is to use a Cornet double-spring forcep (Fig. 2) especially made for holding the cover-glass while staining.) A small drop of water from one of the tumblers is next placed in the centre of the slip with the straight or small-looped needle. (This, of course, is not always necessary, especially if the preparation is being made from a fluid.) The tube (agar we will suppose), containing the culture it is desired to examine, is held also in the left hand between the middle and "ring" fingers, and a very minute portion of the culture is transferred to the drop of water with the sterilized straight needle. If the water becomes slightly turbid, or if a small white speck is seen on the slip after touching the needle-point to the drop, there is sufficient material and the needle should again be sterilized. After cooling the needle return it to the drop and spread the latter about upon the slip. If the drop is small enough evaporation quickly takes place during the spreading, but this may be hastened by holding the glass high above the flame. When the evaporation is complete the result is a scarcely visible, whitish film upon the cover-glass. The slip is next grasped with the forceps, held in the right hand, thoroughly dried high above the flame, and then "fixed" as usual by passing the slip three times through the flame. With the left hand quickly lift a pipetteful of the desired stain and flood the glass to its edges: return the pipette and put the cover-glass for a moment in the lower part of the Bunsen flame until a thin, white steam arises from the fluid; wash in one of the above-mentioned tumblers of water, complete washing in the second and at once invert upon the slide. Pull a strip of filter-paper from the bunch, fold it from end to end, and press it upon the cover-glass and slide, passing the finger-tips over the paper several times. Superfluous water is thus absorbed at once, excepting a very little upon the surface of the cover-slip, which water may quickly be removed with a corner of the folded paper, resting the slide upon the index finger and holding the slip in position with the thumb nail. Finally a drop of cedar-oil completes the preparation, which is immediately examined with the microscope. If the preparation has been properly spread, nearly every field is good; there is no massing of the organisms so as to make it almost impossible to study them carefully except in a few fields; on the contrary, almost every organism stands out very clearly. Such a preparation, including the cleaning of the cover-glass, may be placed under the microscope in less than three minutes. Usually a moment's examination is all that is necessary, but if one desires a longer study care must be taken that the water beneath the slip does not evaporate. Three or four such preparations, depending upon the size of the cover-glasses, may be mounted on one slide.

As before mentioned, by far the greater number of cover-glass preparations are only made for diagnosis, and are then thrown away; it is, therefore, absolutely unnecessary to mount at once in Canada balsam. If, after examination in water, it is desired to preserve any specimen, the procedure is simply as follows: Again holding the slip down with the thumb nail the oil is wiped off with a piece of filter-paper or a cloth moistened with xylol (a bottle of which should be within reach); a drop of water is then placed at the edge of the cover-glass, which is slipped off and dried between folds of filter-paper. After completing the drying over the flame, the preparation is mounted in balsam. The specimen being already known there is, therefore, no need of examining it again until the balsam becomes dry.

A recent method of making and of staining the preparation upon the slide and examining at once in oil without the intervention of a cover-glass, has some advantages and it often saves time. The great advantage of this method is, that four or five different preparations (made exactly as are cover-glass preparations) may be made upon one slide and be stained simultaneously. After washing and thoroughly drying the slide the preparations are ready for examination upon the addition of a drop of oil. Many cover-glasses are thus saved, the slides, which are easily cleaned with a little alcohol, being ready for further use. The great disadvantage of this method is the impracticability of properly mounting permanently, if so desired, any one or more of the specimens thus prepared. If but one preparation is made upon a slide permanent mounting is simple, but, as remarked above, the great advantage of this method lies in the possibility of staining four or five preparations at one time.

An excellent fluid for cleaning slides and cover-glasses, in fact, for cleaning any glassware, is the following:

Water ....50 parts
Alcohol ....45 parts
Ammonia .... 5 parts

The writer has tried many methods and many fluids for cleaning up old balsam or other preparations, but he has never found anything so satisfactory as the above. A small covered vessel of this fluid may be kept upon the desk, and any preparations that are further useless may be placed therein and allowed to remain until one has a leisure hour for cleaning them. In a few days the balsam or the dried material upon the glass or the slide becomes softened or loosened and is easily rubbed off with a cloth; thus covers and slides may be used over and over again.

Another place wherein a little time may be saved is in making plate-cultures. Petri dishes have largely displaced the old-fashioned plates, but the latter may still often be employed to advantage, and much time may be gained, by having a sufficiently large cooling-plate, upon which, under three small bell-jars, the small plates can be cooled. All three plates (for although as a rule only two plates are preserved, it is often wise to keep all three) are then flowed in rapid succession, and while the gelatin is cooling the moist chamber may be prepared. Moreover, it is a useless waste of time to label each tube in writing as the dilutions are being made; it is sufficient simply to mark each tube by twisting a small portion of the cotton-plug into one or two small "ears."

Again much time may be saved by not labelling every tube-culture. It is customary to "carry over" each different culture in the laboratory supply every month. In doing this one generally makes several new cultures, for instance: Two or more cultures in gelatin; two or more in or upon agar; on agar and glycerine; on potatoes, etc. By this procedure one is apt not only to notice the variations of growth in the organism, but runs no risk of also losing one or more altogether by the accidental entrance of some mould or other foreign plant. These new cultures, then, having been made are best placed in a tumbler having a little cotton in the bottom to prevent breakage, placing only cultures of the same organism in one tumbler. It is now absolutely useless to label each tube; writing upon a piece of filter-paper and placing this writing outward within the tumbler is all sufficient.

2. STAINING METHODS.

The following are a few simple methods, in constant use, arranged with special attention to convenience in laboratory work[1]:

I. STAINING BACTERIA IN COVER-GLASS PREPARATIONS WITH WATERY SOLUTIONS OF ANILINE DYES.[2]

1. MAKING THE COVER-GLASS PREPARATIONS.

(a) From Fluid Parts of the Body.—With the sterilized straight or small looped platinum-needle place a small drop of blood or of pus upon the well-cleaned cover-glass and spread it out upon the latter in as even and as thin a film as possible; or, with a sterilized knife, a scraping from the freshly-cut surface of the organ to be examined is spread out in a like manner; or, the cover-glass is pressed directly against the freshly-cut surface of the organ.

(Before cutting an organ burn the surface where the cut is to be made with the flat side of a very hot knife.)

(b) From Pieces of Tissue.—With sterilized forceps pull out a small particle of tissue from the freshly-cut surface of the organ, crush between the forceps, and spread a portion of this crushed tissue substance (with the platinum-needle or the points of the forceps) upon the cover-glass as above directed.

2. "FIXING" THE COVER-GLASS PREPARATION.

To fix the preparation the cover-slip is held in the forceps high above the flame, "butter" side uppermost,

[1] For anthrax, symptomatic anthrax (black-leg), hog cholera, mouse septicæmia, typhoid fever, gonococcus; tetanus, pus organisms, etc., and probably all saprophytic bacteria.

[2] SOLUTIONS OF THE ANILINE DYES: (a) of the dye, 2 parts; water 85 parts; boil from five to ten minutes, and after cooling add 15 parts of 90 per cent. alcohol; mix thoroughly and filter twice. (b) Requisite amounts of concentrated alcoholic solutions of the dyes are diluted ten times with water.

until thoroughly dried. It is then passed three times through the flame at intervals of about one second.

3. STAINING THE COVER-GLASS.

(a) Holding the cover-slip "butter" side up horizontally in the forceps, the glass is flooded to its edges with a pipetteful of the desired staining fluid.

(b) Allow the fluid to remain from one-fourth to one-half a minute upon the slip, or the staining may be hastened by heating the slip until a light steam arises.

(c) Wash the slip in water. If gentian-violet and fuchsin are used it is better if the wash water contains from one-third per cent. to one-fourth per cent. of acetic acid. Afterward, however, wash the slip thoroughly in pure water.

4. EXAMINATION OF THE STAINED COVER-GLASS.

(a) Lay the just washed cover-glass upon a slide ("butter" side down); absorb the superfluous water by placing a folded strip of filter-paper upon both slip and slide, and by lightly running the finger-tips over the same. Holding the cover in place with the thumb nail, remove all moisture from the surface of the cover with a corner of the filter-paper. Examine with the microscope (placing a small drop of cedar-oil in the centre of the cover if desirous of using an oil-immersion lens). Or:

(b) Thoroughly dry the cover-glass first by pressing it between two folds of filter-paper and then by holding it above the flame. Place a small drop of Canada balsam, thinned with xylol, in the centre of the slide and place the cover-slip upon it. Preparations, examined first in water, may then be thus mounted in balsam, after first removing the cedar-oil with filter-paper moistened with xylol, and then removing the cover-glass from the slide.

15

II. STAINING BACTERIA IN SECTIONS WITH WATERY SOLUTIONS OF THE ANILINE DYES.[1]

1. Section from alcohol into water, one minute.

2. In staining fluid,[2] two minutes to five minutes.

3. Decolorize in acidulated water (acetic acid 1:1000), one minute.

4. Wash in eighty per cent. alcohol; then wash and dehydrate in absolute alcohol until no more coloring matter comes away.

5. Clear in oil of cloves, cedar-oil, or oil of origanum.

6. Transfer to the slide, with a spatula or with cigarette paper, and absorb superfluous oil with filter-paper.

7. Bring a drop of xylol-balsam upon the section and place a cover-glass upon it.

[1]For the bacteria mentioned under I.
[2]See I, foot-note 2, a and b.

III. GRAM-GUNTHER METHOD OF STAINING BAC-
TERIA IN SECTIONS.[1]

(A) Without Previous Staining:

1. Section from alcohol into aniline-water-gentian-violet solution,[2] from one to five minutes.

2. Transfer to iodine solution,[3] two minutes. The superfluous staining fluid may first be absorbed with filter-paper.

3. Alcohol, one-half minute.

4. One per cent. hydrochloric acid alcohol, ten seconds.

5. Wash in several watch-glasses of alcohol until entirely decolorized and dehydrated.

6. Cedar-oil or clove-oil.

7. Balsam.

(B) Staining Afterward With a Contrast Color:

1. Section treated as above under A until after decolorization with alcohol, then:

2. From one-fourth to one-half minute in watery Bismarck-brown or Eosin solution.

3. Wash and dehydrate in alcohol.

4. Oil.

5. Balsam.

(C) Staining Previously With a Contrast Color:

1. Section from water to picrocarmine solution,[4] from twenty to thirty minutes.

2. Wash four or five times in fresh water.

3. Alcohol, ten minutes.

4. same as above under A (1 to 7).

[1]Not appropriate for the bacilli of typhoid fever, for glanders, malignant œdema, symptomatic anthrax, the gonococcus, etc., but is appropriate for the bacilli of anthrax, for mouse-septicæmia, tetanus, the micrococcus ascoformans, etc.

[2] (a) Aniline oil ....4 cc
Water.................................100 cc
Mix and filter through previously moistened filter-paper.
Concentrated alc. sol. gentian-violet..........11 cc
This solution remains useful for from three to four weeks.
(b) Saturated watery solution aniline oil, filter; add concentrated alc. solution gentian-violet until a marked metallic film appears on the surface of the fluid.

[3] Iodine .... 1 part.
Iodide of potassium........................2 parts
H_2O.............................300 parts

[4] Picrocarmine solution (Friedlander).
Carmine
Ammonia aa...............................1 part
Water.........................c..........50 parts
To this solution add concentrated watery solution of picric acid until the resulting precipitate no longer dissolves upon stirring. A trace of ammonia added dissolves the precipitate.

19

IV. GRAM METHOD OF STAINING BACTERIA IN COVER-GLASS PREPARATIONS.

1. Hold the cover-glass with forceps, and flood its surface with aniline-water-gentian-violet solution (See III, foot-note 2, a and b). Place glass in a flame until the fluid boils,[1] or stain in the cold from two to five minutes with the same fluid in a watch-glass.

2. Iodine solution (See III, foot-note 3), two minutes.

3. Acid alcohol (HCl. one per cent.), ten seconds.

4. Alcohol until thoroughly decolorized.

5. Contrast stain with water solution of eosin or Bismarck-brown, one minute.

6. Wash in water.

7. Dry and mount.

[1]Boiling the fluid is only necessary when staining the bacillus of tuberculosis.

V. ZIEHL-GABBET METHOD OF STAINING TUBERCLE BACILLI IN COVER-GLASS PREPARATIONS.

(a) 1. Spread a small portion of the material (sputum, cheesy mass, mucus, etc.), that is most likely to contain the bacilli, upon the cover-glass in as thin a layer as possible.

2. Dry and "fix."

3. Flood the glass (held in the forceps) with Ziehl's carbol-fuchsin solution.[1]

4. Boil three or four times and allow the fluid to remain on the glass from one to five minutes. The boiling is accomplished by holding the cover-glass in the lower portion of the Bunsen flame until the staining fluid steams; then slowly raise the glass to the top of the flame and the fluid will boil; immediately lower again and repeat.

5. Wash in water and partially dry the cover-glass with filter-paper.

6. Flood the glass with Gabbet's solution,[2] from one to three minutes, according to the thickness of the preparation and to the intensity of the fuchsin stain.

7. Wash in water; place the cover-slip ("butter" side down) on the slide; absorb the water with filter-paper, etc., and examine; or, to obtain a better contrast, stain (this is no longer the method of Ziehl-Gabbet).

(b) 7. After 6, wash in water.

8. Stain as usual with 2 per cent. methylene-blue (See 1, foot-note 2, a).

9. Wash in water.

10. Mount, etc., or, after 4:

(c) 5. Wash in water.

6. Decolorize in 25 per cent. nitric acid, from ten to thirty seconds.

7. Complete decolorization in alcohol.

8. Wash in water.

9. Stain with methylene-blue, etc., as above (b).

[1] Ziehl's Carbol-fuchsin Solution:
    Fuchsin .... 1 g.
    Alcohol .... 10 cc.
    Carbolic Acid, 5 per cent. .... 100 cc.
Warm to dissolve the fuchsin, and when cool filter.

[2] Gabbet's Solution:
    Methylene-blue .... 1 to 2 g.
    H_2SO_4 25 per cent. .... 100 cc.
Filter.

23

VI. KOCH-EHRLICH METHOD OF STAINING TUBERCLE BACILLI IN COVER-GLASS PREPARATIONS.

1 and 2 same as V (a).

3. Float the cover-glass ("butter" side down) upon Koch-Ehrlich's aniline-water-gentian-violet (methylene-blue or fuchsin) solution,[1] for from twelve to twenty-four hours at room-temperature, or one hour if heated, until a vapor arises.

4. Decolorize in 25 per cent. nitric acid, from ten to thirty seconds.

5. Wash in alcohol until no more color comes away.

6. Contrast stain with a watery solution Bismarck-brown (if fuchsin has been previously used with methylene-blue) one or two minutes.

7. Wash in water and place upon slide, or

8. Dry and mount in balsam.

[1]For preparation of aniline-water-gentian-violet-fuchsin, or methylene blue solutions (See III, foot-note 2, a and b).

VII. KOCH-EHRLICH METHOD OF STAINING TUBERCLE BACILLI IN SECTIONS.

1. Section from alcohol to freshly prepared aniline-water-fuchsin solution,[1] for at least twelve hours at room or incubator temperature.

2. Decolorize in 25 per cent. nitric acid from ten to thirty seconds.

3. Continue decolorization in alcohol until section is pinkish-white.

4. Contrast stain in watery methylene-blue solution one or two minutes.

5. Dehydrate in alcohol.

6. Oil, balsam.

[1]See III, foot-note 2, a and b. Instead of aniline-water-fuchsin solution, aniline-water-gentian-violet, or methylene-blue, may be used, but the latter stains do not seem to be retained so permanently.

VIII. ARENS' METHOD OF STAINING TUBERCLE BACILLI.[1]

(A). IN COVER-GLASS PREPARATIONS.

1. Stain from four to six minutes in chloroform-fuchsin solution.[2]

2. Decolorize in 96 per cent. alcohol + 3 drops HCl to a watch-glass.

3. Wash in water.

4. Contrast stain with methylene-blue, etc.

(B) IN SECTIONS.

1. Sections from alcohol to chloroform-fuchsin solution, four to six minutes.

2. Decolorize as under A 2.

3. Wash in water.

4. Contrast stain, etc.

[1] Recommended for staining these bacilli in fatty substances, milk, etc.

[2] CHLOROFORM-FUCHSIN SOLUTION:
(a) one or two crystals of fuchsin dissolved in from 2 to 3 cc chloroform, or (b) concentrated alcohol solution fuchsin, 3 to 4 drops.

IX. STAINING TUBERCLE BACILLI IN SECTIONS WITH ZIEHL'S CARBOL-FUCHSIN SOLUTION.

(A) ALCOHOL SECTIONS.

1. Stain from ten to twenty minutes in Ziehl's carbol-fuchsin solution (See V, foot-note 1).

2. Same as VII, 2 to 6.

(B) FROZEN SECTIONS.

(a) 1. Sections from salt-solution to 80 or 96 per cent. alcohol for about five minutes to harden. That the section may remain smooth, it is best to transfer it as follows: Lift from the salt-solution with a spatula; drain off superfluous fluid; add 1 to 2 drops of alcohol with the end of a glass rod, and after a moment slip off into alcohol.

2. Same as above under A, or

(b) 1. Sections from salt-solution to water.

2. Harden in corrosive sublimate (1:1000 to 1:500) from one-half to one hour.

3. Wash in water and proceed as above under A.

X. WEIGERT'S FIBRIN OR BACTERIA STAIN IN SECTIONS.

1. Transfer section from water or alcohol to the slide and absorb all the moisture with filter-paper.

2. Flood the section (using a pipette) with aniline-water-gentian-violet solution (See III, foot-note 2, a and b), from one to two minutes, and absorb the stain with filter-paper.

3. Flood the section (using a pipette) with iodine solution (See III, foot-note 3) two minutes, and absorb with filter-paper.

4. Wash the section repeatedly with aniline-xylol[1] until it is nearly decolorized.

5. Wash several times with xylol and as usual absorb with filter-paper.

6. Balsam.

[1] Aniline oil ....2 parts
Xylol ....1 part

XI. STAINING THE GLANDERS BACILLUS.

(A) IN COVER-GLASS PREPARATIONS.

a. LOEFFLER'S OLD METHOD.

1. Flood the cover-glass for three minutes with Loeffler's methylene-blue solution (See XIV, foot-note 2).

2. Heat in the flame until the fluid steams (do not boil).

3. Wash in water.

4. Wash in acetic-acid water (1:100) from five to ten seconds.

5. Wash in water.

6. Mount, etc.

b. LOEFFLER'S NEW METHOD.

1. Flood the glass with alkaline aniline-water-gentian-violet solution,[1] five minutes.

2. Wash in acetic-acid water (1:100) rendered a Rhine-wine-yellow color by the addition of a few drops of tropaeolin (oo) solution.

3. Wash in water, mount, etc.

c. A SIMPLE METHOD.

1. Flood the cover-glass with 2 per cent. gentian-violet solution (See under I, foot-note 2 a).

2. Heat in the flame until the fluid steams well (do not boil), and allow it to stand from one-quarter to one-half minute.

3. Wash in water, mount, etc.

(B) IN SECTIONS.

a. LOEFFLER'S METHOD.

1. Stain for a few minutes in Loeffler's methylene-blue solution (See XIV, foot-note 2).

2. Five seconds in the following solution: Aq. dest., 10cc; concentrated H_2SO_4 2 drops; 5 per cent. oxalic acid, 1 drop.

3. Decolorize and dehydrate in absolute alcohol; oil; balsam.

[1] Alkaline aniline-water-gentian-violet solution (See III, foot-note 2, a, b) mixed with an equal amount of a potash solution (1:10,000), or an equal amount of Liq. Ammon, caustic, half per cent.

b. NONIEWICZ'S METHOD.

1. Section from alcohol to Loeffler's solution (See XIV, foot-note 2), from two to five minutes.

2. Wash in water and transfer to a decolorizing fluid[1], in which thin sections are dipped once beneath the surface, thicker sections remain from three to five seconds.

3. Wash in water.

4. Transfer section to slide and allow to dry thoroughly in the air, or carefully dry over the flame.

5. Balsam.

[1]Acetic acid, ½ per cent...................75 parts.
½ per cent. water tropaeoline (oo) solution..25 parts.

XII. STAINING SPORES, ESPECIALLY ANTHRAX SPORES.

To obtain very beautiful preparations of anthrax spores the following method is recommended: Make hanging-drop cultures in bouillon from the heart's blood of an anthrax mouse (or other experiment animal), using a scarcely-visible amount of blood; place the incubator at 35 to 37 degrees C.; in a few hours the well-known beautiful threads and ropes are formed, and after from twenty-four to forty-eight hours these threads are usually filled with spores (Pl. I, Figs. 1, 2). The cover-glasses are then removed from the slide (first lifting one edge with a knife-blade), dried in the air, the vaseline washed off with xylol, and stained as follows:

1. Fix the dried preparation.

2. Float "butter" side down, on the surface of aniline-water-fuchsin-solution (See III, foot-note 2, a and b, substituting fuchsin for gentian-violet); heat until a delicate vapor arises and continue this for from five to six hours (if much evaporation occurs more aniline-water must be added). It is better to leave the preparation in the dye four or five hours after it has cooled.

3. Decolorize in 25 per cent. HNO_3 about five seconds.

4. Carefully wash in alcohol until no more color comes away, and place for a short time in distilled water.

5. Contrast stain in watery methylene-blue solution, five minutes.

6. Wash carefully in water, mount, etc., and examine. If the preparation is satisfactory:

7. Dry and mount in balsam.

XIII. MOLLER'S METHOD OF STAINING SPORES.

1. Dry and fix the cover-glass preparation.
2. In chloroform, two minutes.
3. Wash in water.
4. In 5 per cent. chromic acid, for a half to two minutes.
5. Water.
6. Flood the glass with Ziehl's carbol-fuchsin solution; boil and keep very hot for one minute.
7. Wash in water.
8. Decolorize in 5 per cent. H_2SO_4 for from five to ten seconds.
9. Wash in water.
10. Stain with methylene-blue.
11. Wash in water, mount, etc.

XIV. STAINING SECTIONS WITH BISMARCK-BROWN, LOEFFLER'S ALKALINE METHYLENE-BLUE, OR WATERY SOLUTIONS OF THE ANILINE DYES.

1. Section from alcohol to water, one minute.

2. Stain with Bismarck-brown,[1] Loeffler's alkaline methylene-blue solution,[2] or with a watery solution of one of the aniline dyes,[3] for ten minutes.

3. Decolorize in a watery solution of acetic acid (1:1000), about one minute.

4. Thoroughly wash in 96 per cent. alcohol, using fresh alcohol several times until no more coloring matter comes away.

5. Oil, balsam, etc.

[1]Bismarck-brown does not stain the bacteria at the same time and is only used to bring out the tissue-structure.

[2]LOEFFLER'S ALKALINE METHYLENE-BLUE.
Concentrated alcohol solution methylene-blue ...30 cc
Watery solution potash (1:1000)...... .... ..100 cc

[3]See I, foot-note 2, a and b.

XV. DOUBLE STAINING OF SECTIONS WITH HEMATOXYLIN AND PICRIC ACID OR EOSIN.

(Only for structure staining, or for staining sections containing actinomyces or the zoogloea masses of the micrococcus ascoformans found in the so-called "scirrhous cord" of the horse).

1. Section from alcohol to Friedlander's hematoxylin[1] solution, from a half-hour to twenty-four hours, according to the strength of the solution.

(It is perhaps best to add to a watch-glass of water or of alum solution (1:250) a sufficient quantity of Friedlander's hematoxylin solution to give the mixture a good red-wine color. In this mixture sections are stained, from one to two hours).

2. Decolorize in 96 per cent. alcohol, and if the section remains too intensely stained, wash alternately in 1 per cent. hydrochloric acid alcohol, and water (or alcohol) r til the section becomes a delicate bluish-red color.

If a single hematoxylin stain only is desired the section is now dehydrated in alcohol, cleared in oil, and mounted in balsam. If, however, a double stain is desired, proceed as follows:

3. DOUBLE STAINING WITH PICRIC ACID.

(a) Transfer the decolorized hematoxylin section to a concentrated alcoholic (96 per cent.) solution of picric acid for a half minute; oil from two to five minutes; balsam; or,

(b) Transfer the decolorized hematoxylin section from alcohol to a watch-glass containing oil of cloves, to which from 10 to 15 drops of a concentrated alcoholic solution of picric acid has been added, five to six minutes; balsam.

4. DOUBLE STAINING WITH EOSIN.

(a) Transfer the decolorized hematoxylin section to a watery solution of eosin,[2] one minute; dehydrate in 96 per cent. alcohol; oil; balsam; or

(b) Transfer the decolorized hematoxylin section from alcohol to a watch-glass containing oil of cloves, to which eight to ten drops of a concentrated alcoholic solution of eosin has been added; balsam.

[1] FRIEDLANDER'S HEMATOXYLIN SOLUTION.
Hematoxylin.
Alum aa..................................2 parts
Alcohol...
Glycerin...
Aq. dest aa..........................100 parts
[2] Add to a watch-glass of water a few drops of a conc. alc. solution of eosin until a distinct eosin-red color is obtained; or mix 1 part of conc. alc. eosin solution with 100 parts of water.

IF THE SECTIONS CONTAIN ACTINOMYCES OR THE ZOOGLOEA MASSES OF THE MICRO-COCCUS ASCOFORMANS.

(SEE PL. II, FIG. 2).

the procedure is as follows:

(a) Stain from one to several hours in a 1 to 2 per cent. watery solution of eosin.

(b) Wash in water and transfer to Friedlander's hematoxylin solution.

(c) Wash in water.

(d) In alcohol.

(e) Decolorize in 1 per cent. hydrochloric acid alcohol, one or two seconds.

(f) Alcohol until dehydrated.

(g) Oil, etc.

47

XVI. TYPICAL METHOD OF STAINING ANTHRAX BACILLI FROM THE BLOOD IN COVER-GLASS PREPARATIONS.

According to Johne the anthrax bacillus in the blood has a typical structure which no other bacillus presents under similar conditions. By this peculiar structure the anthrax bacillus can quickly and absolutely be diagnosed from other large cadaver bacilli often found in the blood of animals from ten to fifteen hours after death and with which bacilli the anthrax bacillus is often confounded.

It is well known that the many organisms are surrounded by a colorless, gelatinous sheath or membrane (often overlooked even when present) similar to the membrane, for instance, frequently seen in some of the higher plants, such as the unicellular algæ. Different environments alter the appearance of this membrane, it some times being very evident and at others scarcely visible or absent in the same organism. For instance, there are several pathogenic bacteria, such as the micrococcus tetragenus, micrococcus ascoformans, and Friedlander's capsule-coccus of pneumonia, which within the body shows a well-defined membrane or capsule, while if grown upon an artificial media this capsule is lost. The same is true of the anthrax bacillus.

If a cover-glass preparation is made from the blood or from the organs of an anthrax animal and is intensely stained with gentian-violet or with fuchsin, there will generally be noticed enormous bacilli of different lengths; with irregular outlines and often with prolonged, rounded swellings at the ends. In such cases it is only with difficulty that the separate cells can be distinguished. If now this preparation is decolorized in 1 to 2 per cent. acetic acid and again be examined a marked alteration will be observed. The bacilli are now seen occuring singly, in pairs, or in distinct chains of varying lengths, still well stained but much smaller than before; their outlines are perfectly regular, except where one is undergoing the process of division, and the ends of the rods are square or more often slightly convex ⊃⊂ never concave ⊐⊏ Surrounding the bacilli, however, is observed a perfectly distinct, colorless membrane. This membrane is apt to be irregular in outline, and its ends are often swollen; it is now very evident that it was this membrane (stained in the first preparation) which caused the apparent size and irregular shapes of the organisms.

It has been suggested that this capsule-like membrane is nothing more than serum clinging to the organisms. This theory cannot, however, be accepted, for not only would such serum be washed away from the bacilli if diluted many times with water (which is not the case),

but serum would also not stain in such a definite manner; moreover, a similar membrane, though much less marked, has been observed in cultures of this organism upon some of our media. We must, therefore, consider this membrane to be a true portion of the bacillus itself and it gives the organism, in the blood of anthrax animals, a very characteristic appearances (Pl. II, Fig. 1), which may be brought out by staining, as follows:

1. Make the cover-glass preparation from the blood, splenic-pulp, etc.

2. Dry and fix.

3. Flood the glass (held in the forceps) with 2 per cent. gentian-violet solution (See I, foot-note 2 a) and stain from a quarter to a half minute.

4. Wash in water.

5. Decolorize in 1 to 2 per cent. acetic acid from five to twenty seconds.

6. Wash in water.

7. Mount, etc.

3. PREPARATION OF NUTRIENT MEDIA.

A. BOUILLON.

1. Add one pound of finely-chopped lean meat to 1000 cc of water, and allow this to stand from twelve to twenty-four hours in a cool place.

2. Strain through cheese-cloth, or a coarse towel, and squeeze in a meat-press, or by twisting the ends of the cloth, until 1000 cc of so-called "meat-" or "flesh-water," are obtained. If less than 1,000 cc are thus obtained, make up the deficiency with fresh water.

3. Add 5g. common salt and dissolve.

4. Add 10g. dried peptone and dissolve.

5. Boil one-quarter hour, either in steam or over an open flame.

6. Make the solution slightly alkaline by the addition of sodium carbonate (saturated solution).

7. Boil from three-quarters to one hour, filter; the filtrate should be clear, if not, add the whites of two eggs, mix rapidly, boil from a quarter to half hour and again filter.[1]

B. BOUILLON (PETRI AND MAASZEN METHOD).

1. Mix meat and water, as above, under A 1, and let it stand for one hour.

2. Heat in water-bath to about 60 degrees C. for three hours.

3. Boil one-half hour.

4. Filter and when cool make slightly alkaline.

5. Add 5g. salt and dissolve.

6. Add 10g. dried Peptone and dissolve.

7. Boil one-quarter hour (best over a free flame).

8. Add glycerine if desired.

9. Filter.

[1] In the preparation of all the peptonized media, it is often the case that the final filtration is not sufficiently clear. This cloudiness is generally due to the fine particles of matter suspended in the fluid. If egg albumen is now added, and the solution is again boiled, these particles are generally caught in the coagulum, and they can be removed with the filter. It is, perhaps, a good practice always to add the eggs before the last boiling, thus avoiding a second filtration. Even after every precaution has been taken, it sometimes seems impossible to obtain a perfectly clear filtrate; in such cases, the repeated addition of eggs and boiling are recommended; in the case of bouillon, the particles will sink to the bottom on cooling, and, as a rule, may then be filtered off.

C. GELATIN.

1. Make meat-water as above, under A 1 and 2.
2. Salt, 5g.
3. Peptone, 10g.
4. Gelatin, 100g.   -
5. Heat in water-bath to 50 degrees until the gelatin is dissolved.
6. Make slightly alkline.
7. Boil three-quarters to one hour.[1]
8. Filter.

D. AGAR-AGAR.

1. Make bouillon (See A and B).
2. Add 10 to 20 g. agar-agar, finely cut up.
3. Boil until the agar is dissolved (five to eight hours).
4. Neutralize if necessary and add glycerin if desired.
5. Boil from three-quarters to one hour.
6. Filter (filtration is often rapid at room-temperature, but if it should occur slowly the agar must be filtered in steam or in a hot-water filter).

E. AGAR-AGAR GELATIN.

This medium is prepared as indicated above, using, however, only 7.5g. of agar, and, when this is dissolved, adding 50g. of gelatin.

F. PREPARING THE PEPTONE MEDIA WITH LIEBIG'S MEAT EXTRACT.

Instead of using chopped meat, Liebig's Meat Extract may be substituted in the proportion of from 3 to 5 grammes to the litre of water.

G. BLOOD-SERUM.

(Ascitic and hydrocele fluid often contain too little albumen to admit of congulation. Such fluids should therefore be tested by boiling before tubing.)

1. Collect the blood in large jars, which can be closed tightly, and close the jars.
2. In about fifteen minutes, or after clotting has begun, pass a sterilized glass rod around the clot, between its surface and the wall of the jar, thus breaking up the glass adhesions, which prevent the clot from sinking.
3. Again close the jars and place them in an ice-chest, for from twenty-four to forty-eight hours.

[1] One must be cautioned against too long boiling of the solution, since this lowers the solidifying point of the gelatin.

4. Draw off serum with sterilized pipette and run into test-tubes.

5. Place tubes in blood-serum sterilizer and heat to 68 or 70 degrees C. for one hour on five successive days.

6. Place tubes in the apparatus for solidifying blood-serum and heat to 75 or 80 degrees C., until the serum is coagulated.

H.   BLOOD-SERUM (QUICK METHOD.)

(Serum made in the following manner is, as a rule, more opaque than that prepared as indicated above; but for all practical purposes it is admirable. Much time and annoyance are saved, and imperfect sterilization, by means common by the other method, is avoided).

1-4 See G.

5. Place the tubes in the serum sterilizer and heat at once to 90 or 95 degrees C. for one hour or more.

6. Place the tubes (in an inclined position) in the steam sterilizer for one hour or more.

(It is advisable not to allow the temperature in the steam sterilizer to run too high or bubbles may result in the solid serum. With the Arnold steam sterilizer, the inside cover may be left off, or with other sterilizers, full gas pressure need not be used.)

7. Place the tubes in baskets as usual, and steam for from fifteen to thirty minutes on two successive days.

4. IMBEDDING TISSUES FOR CUTTING SECTIONS.

A. IMBEDDING IN CELLOIDIN.

1. Transfer the hardened tissue from alcohol to equal parts of alcohol and ether, twelve hours or longer.

2. Into thin celloidin, twelve hours or longer.

3. Into thicker celloidin, thirteen hours or longer.

4. Into thick celloidin (that is, so thick that the specimens but slowly sink to the bottom), twelve hours or longer.

5. Place specimen with as much celloidin as possible clinging to it upon cork, a small block of wood, or, best, a block of vulcanized fibre.[1] With a glass rod add several layers of the thick celloidin until the specimen is quite surrounded, especially toward its base, with perhaps one-eighth inch of celloidin. Allow it to remain in the air until a sufficiently thick film forms on the outside, then

6. Into 50 to 75 per cent. alcohol (the celloidin must be beneath the surface of the fluid) to harden; or harden quickly by dropping it into chloroform, and after a few minutes place in alcohol (75 per cent.).

7. Cut in alcohol.

B. IMBEDDING IN CELLOIDIN AND PARAFFIN.

1—4. See above under A.

5. Drop into chloroform and keep immersed (by means of a small net loosely attached to a wire frame, for instance) from six to eight hours.

6. Place in melted paraffin[2], one to two days; or better, place in a bottle of melted paraffin kept at 55 to 58 degrees C. in a water-bath, attach a suction pump[3] and pump until a few, or no more, bubbles come away from the tissues, from one to three hours.

[1]This may be obtained from the Vulcanized Fibre Co., Wilmington, Del., and, when cut into small blocks, is admirable for mounting tissues imbedded in celloidin. One may write with a pencil upon the blocks and they readily sink in fluids, thus saving much trouble.

[2]Hard and soft paraffin are mixed in such proportion that the melting point of the combined mass is about 52 degrees C.

[3]A Chapman water-pump is the simplest and best to use for this purpose.

7. Imbed in paraffin.[1]

8. Cut with a Minot microtome. Such sections may be placed in a box and they will keep indefinitely. Before staining—

9. Sections into chloroform or benzole to dissolve paraffin, using two watch-glasses of the fluid.

10. Into absolute alcohol, using two watch-glasses of the fluid.

11. Stain.

[1]For this purpose cheap and very satisfactory paraffin moulds may be made from four pieces of heavy type-metal (brass is in commoner use, but is more expensive). These pieces need not be fastened together, thus permitting moulds of different sizes to be formed. Small pasteboard boxes may also be used. These pieces of metal are placed upon a glass plate, a mould of the desired size is formed and filled with melted paraffin, first, however, smearing the surfaces, which are later to come in contact with the paraffin, with the glycerin. Soon a thin, semi-solid layer of paraffin forms at the bottom of the mould, and the material to be cut is then placed into and held in any position desired by this layer. When the paraffin has cooled so that a thin film or crust has formed on its surface, immerse the mould and all in cold water. The block of paraffin is thus quickly hardened and the mould can almost immediately be removed.

PLATE I.

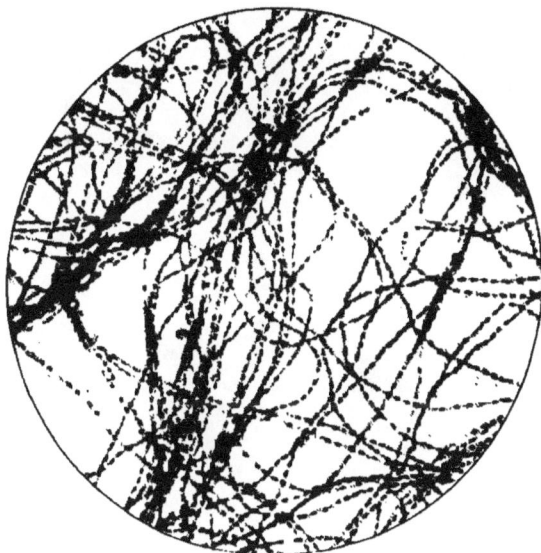

FIG. 1.—Anthrax bacilli: hanging-drop culture from blood, showing threads and spores (x ca. 700).

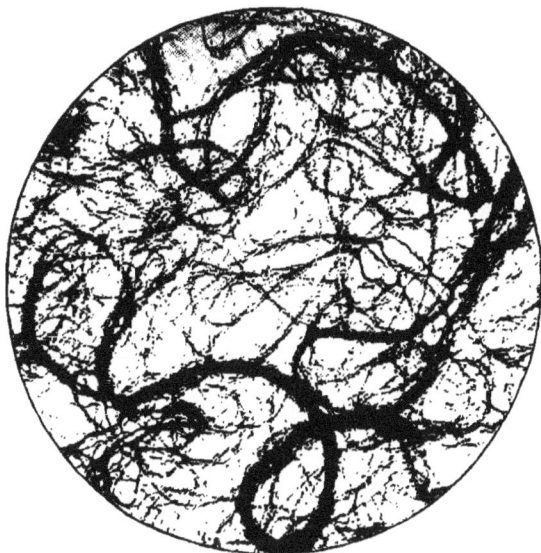

FIG. 2.—Anthrax from hanging-drop culture from blood, showing threads and ropes (x 130).

PLATE II.

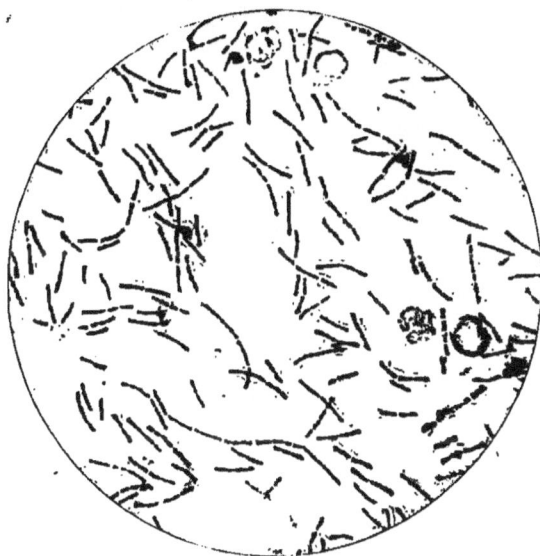

FIG 1.—Anthrax bacilli from spleen of a mouse.

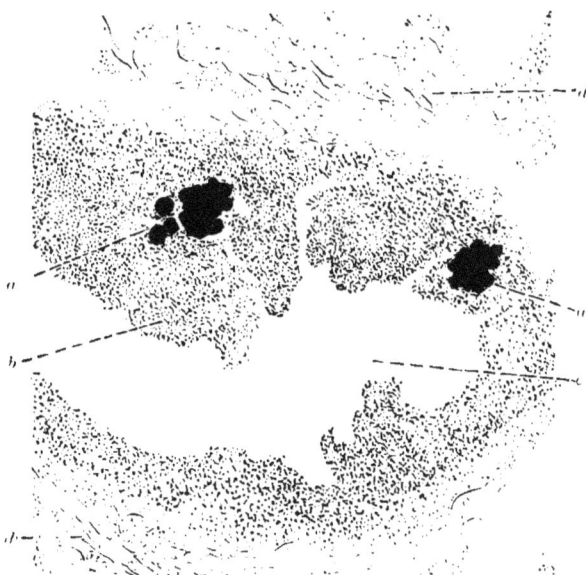

FIG 2.—Section of "myko-fibrom" from the spermatic cord of a horse (x ca 50): *a*. grape-like clusters of zoöglœa (containing cocci not visible) ; *b*, cellular centre, consisting of pus and some lymphoid cells ; *c*, space from which cells have fallen out ; *d*, fibrous stroma (stained by method xv. 5).

www.ingramcontent.com/pod-product-compliance
Lightning Source LLC
Chambersburg PA
CBHW022006190326
41519CB00010B/1408